7 PROVEN WAYS TO STAY HEALTHY

A Holistic Approach to Your Well-being

BY

James Clifford

TABLE OF CONTENTS

INTRODUCTION

In the pursuit of a thriving and fulfilling life, the concept of holistic health has emerged as a guiding principle, emphasizing the interconnectedness of various aspects of our well-being. This chapter serves as a foundational exploration into the essence of holistic health, providing a lens through which we can view our health as a comprehensive and integrated experience.

Defining Holistic Health:

Holistic health extends beyond the absence of illness; it encompasses a dynamic equilibrium of the physical, mental, emotional, and spiritual dimensions. It recognizes that these facets of our being are interdependent, and achieving true health involves addressing each aspect in harmony. Holistic health, therefore, advocates for a balanced and synergistic approach to well-being, considering the whole person rather than isolated symptoms or conditions.

Overview of the Seven Proven Ways to Stay Healthy:

Within the realm of holistic health, we embark on a journey guided by seven proven ways to stay healthy. Each of these strategies contributes to a comprehensive understanding of health, promoting a state of equilibrium that fosters vitality and resilience. From the choices we make in our nutrition to the mindful practices that shape our mental well-being, these seven pillars serve as a roadmap toward a healthier, more fulfilling life.

Importance of a Well-Rounded Approach to Well-being:

While modern medicine excels at addressing specific ailments, a well-rounded approach to well-being acknowledges that health is a multifaceted tapestry. Rather than isolating symptoms and treating them in isolation, holistic health embraces the idea that the mind, body, and spirit are intricately interconnected. By recognizing and nurturing this interconnectedness, individuals can cultivate a state of balance that promotes optimal health and a higher quality of life.

This book unfolds as a comprehensive guide to navigating the terrain of holistic health, offering practical insights and evidence-based strategies to empower you on your journey. As we delve into each of the seven proven ways to stay healthy, remember that the pursuit of well-being is not a one-size-fits-all endeavor. Rather, it is an individual and evolving path that encourages self-discovery and a deeper understanding of the intricate tapestry that is your health. Join us in exploring the transformative potential of holistic health, and let this journey be a catalyst for positive change in your life.

CHAPTER 1:

THE POWER OF NUTRITION

In the quest for holistic health, nutrition emerges as a cornerstone, wielding a profound influence on our overall well-being. This chapter delves into the transformative power of nutrition, unraveling the intricate relationship between what we consume and the vitality we experience.

Exploring the Impact of a Balanced Diet on Health:

The adage "you are what you eat" holds a profound truth. A balanced diet, rich in essential nutrients, is the bedrock of good health. This section examines the far-reaching impact of a well-rounded and nourishing diet on various aspects of our physical and mental well-being. From bolstering the immune system to supporting cognitive function, the influence of nutrition on our health is multifaceted.

A balanced diet not only provides the necessary fuel for our bodies but also plays a pivotal role in preventing chronic diseases and maintaining optimal organ function. By understanding the fundamental principles of balanced nutrition, we empower ourselves to make informed dietary choices that resonate with our body's needs.

Nutrient-Rich Foods for Optimal Well-being:

The journey to holistic health involves embracing a palette of nutrient-rich foods that serve as potent allies in our pursuit of well-being. This section guides readers through the vibrant world of fruits, vegetables, whole grains, lean proteins, and healthy fats. Each of these food categories contributes unique vitamins, minerals, and antioxidants, fostering a symphony of nutrients essential for robust health.

Exploration of nutrient-dense foods goes beyond a mere list of dietary recommendations; it illuminates the profound impact these choices have on our energy levels, mood, and long-term health. By incorporating a variety of nutrient-rich foods into our meals, we not only savor a diverse array of flavors but also provide our bodies with the tools needed for optimal functioning.

Tailoring Your Diet to Individual Needs:

Recognizing the diversity of human physiology, this section emphasizes the importance of tailoring our diets to individual needs. Factors such as age, gender, activity level, and underlying health conditions influence our nutritional requirements. Understanding these nuances empowers individuals to create a personalized approach to nutrition that aligns with their unique biological makeup.

Consulting with healthcare professionals or nutritionists can further refine this process, providing personalized guidance on dietary choices. By acknowledging and respecting the individuality of our nutritional needs, we embark on a journey towards a sustainable and nourishing relationship with food.

As we navigate the landscape of nutrition, let us embark on a mindful exploration of the foods that fuel our bodies and minds. Through informed choices and a commitment to nourishing ourselves with intention, we unlock the transformative power of nutrition on our holistic health journey.

CHAPTER 2:

EXERCISE FOR A HEALTHY BODY AND MIND

Physical activity is a dynamic force that shapes not only the contours of our bodies but also the landscape of our mental and emotional well-being. In this chapter, we unravel the multifaceted dimensions of exercise, exploring its diverse forms, the art of crafting a personalized fitness routine, and the profound impact it holds on the intricate tapestry of our mental health.

Understanding the Different Types of Exercises:

Exercise is not a one-size-fits-all endeavor; it encompasses a spectrum of activities, each offering unique benefits. This section provides an insightful exploration into various types of exercises, including cardiovascular workouts, strength training, flexibility exercises, and mind-body practices like yoga and tai chi. Understanding the diverse range of exercises allows individuals to tailor their routines to encompass a holistic approach to fitness.

From the invigorating rush of a morning jog to the meditative flow of yoga, each type of exercise contributes to overall well-being in distinctive ways. By embracing a variety of activities, individuals can create a balanced exercise regimen that not only promotes physical health but also caters to personal preferences and goals.

Creating a Personalized Fitness Routine:

Crafting an effective and sustainable fitness routine involves aligning exercise with individual preferences, goals, and lifestyle. This section provides practical guidance on developing a personalized fitness plan, considering factors such as fitness level, time constraints, and specific health objectives. Whether aiming for weight management, strength building, or overall vitality, a personalized routine ensures that exercise becomes an integral and enjoyable part of daily life.

Moreover, the chapter delves into the importance of incorporating both aerobic and anaerobic exercises for a well-rounded fitness approach. Balancing cardiovascular workouts with strength and flexibility training enhances overall physical resilience, contributing to a robust and adaptable body.

Benefits of Regular Physical Activity for Mental Health:

The connection between physical activity and mental well-being is profound and transformative. This section explores the intricate ways in which exercise positively influences mental health, including the release of endorphins, improved cognitive function, stress reduction, and enhanced mood. Regular physical activity has been linked to a decreased risk of depression, anxiety, and other mental health disorders.

As we embark on the journey of holistic health, let us recognize the invaluable role that exercise plays in sculpting not only our physical bodies but also nurturing the resilience and vitality of our minds. By embracing the diversity of exercise options and tailoring routines to individual needs, we harness the power of movement as a potent force for holistic well-being.

CHAPTER 3:

THE ROLE OF SLEEP IN WELL-BEING

In the rhythmic dance of life, sleep emerges as a crucial partner, influencing our physical health, mental clarity, and emotional resilience. This chapter delves into the profound significance of quality sleep, guiding readers through the elements that contribute to a restful night and the cultivation of optimal well-being.

Importance of Quality Sleep:

Sleep is more than a temporary retreat from daily activities; it is a fundamental cornerstone of well-being. This section explores the physiological and psychological importance of quality sleep. Adequate and restorative sleep is linked to enhanced immune function, improved memory consolidation, emotional regulation, and overall physical recovery. Understanding the transformative power of sleep invites individuals to prioritize this essential aspect of health.

The chapter emphasizes the role of sleep in promoting longevity, reducing the risk of chronic diseases, and optimizing cognitive performance. Through a comprehensive exploration of the multifaceted benefits of quality sleep, readers gain insights into the profound impact that sleep has on their holistic health.

Creating a Sleep-Friendly Environment:

Crafting an environment conducive to quality sleep is an art that involves both the physical and sensory aspects of our surroundings. This section provides practical tips on designing a sleep-friendly space, including considerations such as room temperature, lighting, and noise levels. Creating a comfortable and calming sleep sanctuary enhances the likelihood of entering restorative sleep cycles.

Exploring the impact of technology on sleep hygiene, this chapter also offers insights into the importance of unplugging from screens before bedtime. By acknowledging the role of environmental factors in sleep quality, individuals can take proactive steps to transform their bedrooms into havens of tranquility.

Tips for Improving Sleep Hygiene:

Sleep hygiene encompasses a set of practices that contribute to healthy sleep patterns. This section offers a comprehensive guide to improving sleep hygiene, covering aspects such as establishing a consistent sleep schedule, cultivating a pre-sleep routine, and moderating caffeine and alcohol intake. Practical tips for managing stress and anxiety before bedtime are also explored, recognizing the role of a calm and focused mind in promoting quality sleep.

Moreover, the chapter delves into the importance of addressing sleep disorders and seeking professional guidance when necessary. By incorporating evidence-based strategies for improving sleep hygiene into daily life, individuals can unlock the transformative potential of restful and rejuvenating sleep.

As we explore the role of sleep in our holistic well-being, let us embrace the notion that a good night's sleep is not just a luxury but an indispensable investment in our health. By understanding the nuances of quality sleep, creating sleep-friendly environments, and adopting effective sleep hygiene practices, we pave the way for a vibrant and resilient life.

Stress Management Techniques:

CHAPTER 4:

STRESS MANAGEMENT TECHNIQUES

Stress, an omnipresent companion in our modern lives, has profound implications for our health and well-being. This chapter is a journey into the realm of stress management, exploring the effects of chronic stress, introducing mindfulness and meditation practices as powerful tools, and providing insights on seamlessly integrating stress management into our daily routines.

Recognizing the Effects of Chronic Stress:

Chronic stress is more than an occasional rush of tension; it's a pervasive force that can impact every facet of our lives. This section delves into the physiological and psychological effects of prolonged stress, from elevated cortisol levels to impaired immune function. Recognizing these effects is the first step toward understanding the urgency of incorporating stress management techniques into our daily lives.

Through real-life examples and relatable scenarios, readers gain insights into the ways chronic stress can manifest, affecting mental clarity, emotional well-being, and physical health. By acknowledging the impact of stress, individuals are empowered to take proactive steps toward resilience and balance.

Mindfulness and Meditation Practices:

Mindfulness and meditation emerge as potent antidotes to the chaos of daily life. This section introduces readers to the transformative practices of mindfulness and meditation, exploring their roots, principles, and practical applications. Mindfulness, the art of being present in the moment without judgment, and meditation, a focused practice that cultivates a calm and centered mind, provide valuable tools for navigating the complexities of stress.

Guided exercises and step-by-step instructions demystify the practice of mindfulness and meditation, making them accessible to individuals at any experience level. By embracing these techniques, readers embark on a journey of self-discovery, learning to observe their thoughts, emotions, and stressors with greater clarity and equanimity.

Integrating Stress Management into Daily Life:

Effective stress management is not an isolated event; it's a seamless integration into the fabric of our daily lives. This section offers practical strategies for weaving stress management into the tapestry of our routines. From micro-moments of mindfulness during hectic days to carving out dedicated time for meditation, the chapter explores a spectrum of approaches that cater to diverse lifestyles.

The importance of establishing healthy boundaries, practicing self-compassion, and fostering a supportive environment is emphasized. Through realistic and adaptable techniques, readers discover how to infuse their days with moments of calm, ultimately building resilience in the face of life's inevitable stressors.

As we navigate the landscape of stress, let us not only recognize its effects but also embrace the transformative potential of stress management techniques. By integrating mindfulness, meditation, and practical stress-reducing strategies into our daily lives, we empower ourselves to navigate life's challenges with grace and resilience.

CHAPTER 5

HYDRATION FOR VITALITY

In the mosaic of health and well-being, hydration stands as a fundamental and often overlooked pillar. This chapter delves into the significance of proper hydration, offering insights into water intake recommendations, and exploring the art of balancing beverages to foster not just quenched thirst but overall vitality.

The Significance of Proper Hydration:

Water, the elixir of life, plays a central role in maintaining optimal bodily functions. This section explores the profound significance of proper hydration, elucidating its impact on cellular health, digestion, temperature regulation, and cognitive function. Readers will gain an understanding of how hydration is intricately linked to physical performance, detoxification processes, and overall vitality.

The chapter also explores the signs of dehydration, emphasizing the importance of listening to our bodies and recognizing when they signal the need for replenishment. By understanding the far-reaching effects of hydration on our well-being, individuals can cultivate a mindful and proactive approach to meeting their body's fluid needs.

Water Intake Recommendations:

How much water is enough? This section provides practical guidance on water intake recommendations, considering factors such as age, climate, physical activity, and individual health conditions. It delves into the concept of thirst as a reliable indicator of hydration needs and dispels common myths surrounding water consumption.

By demystifying the daily requirement for water intake and offering tips on staying adequately hydrated throughout the day, readers gain actionable insights into maintaining optimal fluid balance. Understanding that hydration is not a one-size-fits-all proposition allows individuals to tailor their intake to their unique circumstances.

Balancing Beverages for Overall Health:

While water is the cornerstone of hydration, this section explores the broader landscape of beverages and their impact on health. From herbal teas to infused waters and hydrating foods, the chapter provides a holistic view of how various fluids contribute to overall well-being. It also addresses the potential pitfalls of sugary and caffeinated beverages, offering strategies for moderation and healthier alternatives.

The chapter emphasizes the importance of mindful beverage choices, considering not only hydration needs but also the nutritional content of different drinks. By balancing the variety of fluids consumed, individuals can nourish their bodies while staying adequately hydrated, fostering a sustainable and health-conscious approach to beverage choices.

As we delve into the depths of hydration for vitality, let us recognize water as a source of life and energy. By understanding the significance of proper hydration, embracing personalized water intake recommendations, and balancing a spectrum of health-conscious beverages, we unlock the door to a well-hydrated and vibrant existence.

CHAPTER 6

NURTURING SOCIAL CONNECTIONS

In the tapestry of well-being, social connections form a vibrant thread, weaving together the fabric of our mental, emotional, and physical health. This chapter explores the profound impact of social relationships on overall well-being, provides insights into building and maintaining meaningful connections, and offers strategies for combating the pervasive sense of loneliness.

Impact of Social Relationships on Well-being:

The intricate dance of human connections has far-reaching effects on our holistic health. This section delves into the profound impact of social relationships, examining how they influence emotional resilience, mental clarity, and even physical health. Research consistently demonstrates that strong social ties are linked to lower stress levels, improved mood, and a reduced risk of chronic diseases.

Readers will gain an understanding of the physiological mechanisms through which social connections affect the body, from the release of oxytocin, the "bonding hormone," to the role of social support in mitigating the effects of stress. Acknowledging the interconnected nature of our well-being with the quality of our social relationships encourages individuals to prioritize and nurture these connections.

Building and Maintaining Meaningful Connections:

Creating and sustaining meaningful connections is an art that requires intention and effort. This section provides practical insights into the dynamics of building and maintaining relationships that contribute positively to well-being. From fostering empathy and effective communication to cultivating shared interests and experiences, readers will discover actionable strategies for deepening the quality of their social connections.

The chapter explores the role of vulnerability in forging authentic relationships, encouraging individuals to be genuine and open in their interactions. Through relatable anecdotes and guidance, readers are empowered to take proactive steps in creating a social network that uplifts and supports them in their journey towards well-being.

Strategies for Combating Loneliness:

Loneliness, an all too common facet of modern life, can have detrimental effects on mental and physical health. This section addresses the nuances of loneliness and offers practical strategies for combatting its pervasive grip. From seeking out community groups and volunteer opportunities to leveraging technology for virtual connections, readers will find a toolkit of approaches to alleviate loneliness and foster a sense of belonging.

The chapter also explores the importance of self-reflection and self-compassion in navigating periods of loneliness. By recognizing that loneliness is a universal experience and actively engaging in strategies to overcome it, individuals can transform their relationship with solitude and build a network of connections that enhance their overall well-being.

As we delve into the realm of nurturing social connections, let us recognize the transformative power of human relationships. By understanding the impact of social ties, actively building meaningful connections, and employing strategies to combat loneliness, individuals can cultivate a social landscape that enriches their lives and contributes to their holistic well-being.

CHAPTER 7

INTEGRATING HOLISTIC HABITS INTO DAILY LIFE

In the hustle and bustle of modern living, the seamless integration of holistic habits into our daily routines becomes an art, paving the way for sustained well-being. This chapter explores the art of creating a holistic wellness routine, offers practical tips for individuals with busy schedules, and unveils the keys to making lifestyle changes that stand the test of time.

Creating a Holistic Wellness Routine:

Holistic wellness is not an isolated endeavor but a tapestry woven through consistent habits. This section guides readers in the creation of a holistic wellness routine that encompasses the key pillars of well-being. From morning rituals that set a positive tone for the day to evening practices that promote relaxation, the chapter offers insights into building a comprehensive routine that nourishes the mind, body, and spirit.

Readers will discover the transformative potential of incorporating elements such as mindfulness, exercise, proper nutrition, and self-care into their daily schedules. The emphasis is on creating a routine that is not only effective but also sustainable over the long term, contributing to a life of balance and vitality.

Practical Tips for Busy Schedules:

For those navigating demanding schedules, the challenge lies in finding realistic and manageable ways to infuse holistic habits into daily life. This section provides practical tips tailored to busy lifestyles, recognizing the importance of adaptability and efficiency. From micro-moments of mindfulness during work breaks to incorporating short, effective workouts, readers will gain insights into maximizing the impact of holistic habits within the constraints of a hectic schedule.

The chapter also explores the concept of time management, encouraging individuals to identify priorities and allocate time mindfully to self-care practices. By recognizing that even small, consistent efforts can yield significant results, readers can overcome the barriers of a busy schedule and embrace holistic well-being.

Making Sustainable Lifestyle Changes:

Creating lasting change is a journey that requires commitment and resilience. This section unravels the keys to making lifestyle changes that endure, emphasizing the importance of gradual progress and self-compassion. By setting realistic goals, understanding personal motivations, and celebrating small victories, individuals can lay the foundation for sustainable and transformative lifestyle changes.

The chapter explores the role of accountability and social support in fostering lasting habits. It also provides strategies for overcoming setbacks and adapting to evolving circumstances, recognizing that the journey to holistic well-being is dynamic and requires a flexible approach.

As we navigate the terrain of integrating holistic habits into daily life, let us embrace the notion that well-being is a journey, not a destination. By crafting a holistic wellness routine, incorporating practical tips into busy schedules, and making sustainable lifestyle changes, individuals can embark on a transformative path towards lasting health, balance, and vitality.

29

CHAPTER 8

THE MIND-BODY CONNECTION

In the intricate dance of well-being, the mind and body are not separate entities but interconnected aspects of our holistic health. This chapter delves into the profound interplay between mental and physical well-being, introduces practices for cultivating a positive mindset, and unravels the transformative influence of the mind on overall health and vitality.

Exploring the Interplay Between Mental and Physical Health:

The mind and body share a dynamic relationship, each influencing the other in ways that shape our overall health. This section explores the interconnected nature of mental and physical well-being, delving into the ways in which stress, emotions, and thought patterns can impact the body. Readers will gain insights into the physiological mechanisms through which mental health influences immune function, hormonal balance, and even recovery from illness.

Understanding the mind-body connection lays the groundwork for a holistic approach to health, recognizing that mental well-being is not just a byproduct but a cornerstone of overall vitality. By acknowledging the interplay between mental and physical health, individuals can cultivate a deeper understanding of their well-being and embrace practices that foster harmony between mind and body.

Practices for Cultivating a Positive Mindset:

A positive mindset is not merely an optimistic outlook; it is a powerful force that shapes our experiences and influences our health. This section introduces practices for cultivating a positive mindset, offering actionable strategies for shifting thought patterns and fostering resilience in the face of life's challenges. From gratitude exercises to affirmations and mindfulness, readers will discover a toolkit of practices that contribute to a more optimistic and empowered mental state.

The chapter explores the role of self-talk and cognitive reframing in shaping perceptions and emotional responses. By adopting practices that nurture a positive mindset, individuals can harness the transformative potential of their thoughts, contributing to enhanced mental well-being and overall life satisfaction.

Harnessing the Mind's Influence on Overall Well-being:

The mind holds a profound influence on the trajectory of our health and vitality. This section delves into the ways in which thoughts, beliefs, and attitudes can impact stress resilience, immune function, and even the body's ability to heal. The chapter explores the concept of psychoneuroimmunology, highlighting the interconnectedness of psychological factors with the nervous and immune systems.

Readers will gain insights into the mind's role in shaping lifestyle choices, influencing habits, and contributing to the prevention of chronic diseases. By recognizing the mind's influence on overall well-being, individuals can become active participants in their health journey, adopting practices that not only enhance mental health but also contribute to a resilient and vibrant life.

As we navigate the profound terrain of the mind-body connection, let us embrace the transformative potential that lies within our thoughts and emotions. By exploring the interplay between mental and physical health, cultivating a positive mindset, and harnessing the mind's influence on overall well-being, individuals can unlock the keys to a more integrated and flourishing life.

The chapter emphasizes the importance of self-compassion and the language we use internally. By adopting practices that foster positivity, individuals can harness the mind's potential to shape their experiences, relationships, and overall quality of life.

Harnessing the Mind's Influence on Overall Well-being:

The mind, as a silent architect, plays a pivotal role in shaping the trajectory of our overall well-being. This section delves into the profound ways in which the mind influences health, from stress management to the prevention of chronic diseases. The chapter explores the emerging field of psychoneuroimmunology, unraveling the intricate connections between psychological factors, the nervous system, and the immune system.

Readers will gain insights into the mind's role in lifestyle choices and habits, understanding how it can be a powerful ally in fostering positive health behaviors. By recognizing the mind's influence on overall well-being, individuals become empowered co-creators of their health journey, adopting practices that not only enhance mental resilience but also contribute to a flourishing and balanced life.

As we journey into the exploration of the mind-body connection, let us embrace the transformative potential inherent in understanding and nurturing this profound relationship. Through practices that cultivate a positive mindset and by harnessing the mind's influence on overall well-being, individuals can embark on a path toward a more integrated, vibrant, and fulfilling existence.

CHAPTER 9
GOAL SETTING FOR HEALTH

In the pursuit of well-being, setting and achieving health goals becomes a compass guiding individuals toward a life of vitality and balance. This chapter explores the art of setting realistic health goals, developing step-by-step action plans, and embracing a process of monitoring progress and celebrating achievements.

Setting Realistic Health Goals:

Effective goal setting is a cornerstone of any successful health journey. This section guides readers in the art of setting realistic and attainable health goals. By considering personal aspirations, motivations, and current health status, individuals can craft goals that are both inspiring and achievable.

The chapter delves into the importance of specificity and clarity in goal formulation, encouraging individuals to define not just what they want to achieve but also why it matters to them. By aligning health goals with personal values and priorities, individuals set the stage for a meaningful and sustainable journey towards well-being.

Developing a Step-by-Step Action Plan:

A well-defined goal is a destination, and an action plan is the roadmap that charts the journey. This section provides practical insights into developing a step-by-step action plan that transforms health goals into actionable and manageable tasks. From identifying key milestones to breaking down larger objectives into smaller, more achievable steps, readers will discover strategies for turning aspirations into tangible actions.

The chapter explores the importance of flexibility and adaptability in action planning, recognizing that life is dynamic, and adjustments may be necessary. By developing a roadmap that is both structured and adaptable, individuals enhance their capacity to navigate the twists and turns of their health journey.

Monitoring Progress and Celebrating Achievements:

The journey toward health is not a linear path; it's a tapestry woven with progress, setbacks, and victories. This section introduces the concept of monitoring progress as an integral part of goal achievement. From tracking measurable outcomes to reflecting on the emotional and physical changes, readers gain insights into the importance of self-awareness and self-reflection.

Celebrating achievements, both big and small, is a vital component of sustaining motivation and momentum. The chapter explores the art of acknowledging progress, fostering a positive mindset, and using achievements as stepping stones for future goals. By recognizing and celebrating successes, individuals infuse their health journey with a sense of accomplishment and motivation.

As we embark on the chapter of goal setting for health, let us embrace the transformative power of aspirations and the practicality of action plans. Through realistic goal setting, thoughtful action planning, and a commitment to monitoring progress and celebrating achievements, individuals pave the way for a life of sustained health, fulfillment, and flourishing well-being.

CHAPTER 10

SELF-CARE STRATEGIES FOR A HEALTHIER YOU

Importance of self-care in maintaining well-being

Designing a personalized self-care routine

Balancing self-care with other life commitments

In the whirlwind of daily life, self-care emerges as a sanctuary—an intentional and nourishing practice that fuels overall well-being. This chapter explores the paramount importance of self-care, guides readers in designing personalized self-care routines, and unveils the art of balancing self-care with other life commitments.

Importance of Self-Care in Maintaining Well-being:

Self-care is not a luxury; it is a fundamental investment in one's health and vitality. This section delves into the profound significance of self-care in maintaining overall well-being. From managing stress to enhancing mental resilience, self-care practices are integral to preventing burnout and fostering a life of balance.

The chapter explores the physiological and psychological benefits of self-care, shedding light on how intentional acts of self-nurturing contribute to emotional equilibrium, physical health, and improved relationships. By understanding the role of self-care in the holistic landscape of well-being, individuals can prioritize and integrate these practices into their daily lives.

Designing a Personalized Self-Care Routine:

Self-care is a deeply personal journey, requiring an intentional and customized approach. This section provides practical insights into designing a personalized self-care routine that resonates with individual preferences, needs, and lifestyles. From mindful practices like meditation and journaling to physical activities and creative pursuits, readers will discover a spectrum of self-care options that align with their unique well-being goals.

The chapter encourages a holistic view of self-care, encompassing not only physical practices but also emotional and mental well-being. By tailoring a routine that addresses diverse aspects of self-nurturing, individuals can create a sustainable and fulfilling self-care practice.

Balancing Self-Care with Other Life Commitments:

In a world filled with responsibilities and commitments, finding the balance between self-care and other obligations is an art. This section explores strategies for harmonizing self-care with work, family, and social commitments. It provides insights into time management, boundary setting, and communication, empowering individuals to navigate the complexities of a busy life while still prioritizing their well-being.

The chapter emphasizes the importance of self-advocacy and the role of self-care in enhancing one's capacity to fulfill other responsibilities. By recognizing that self-care is not selfish but a necessary foundation for sustained productivity and happiness, individuals can cultivate a balanced and integrated approach to life.

As we delve into the chapter on self-care strategies, let us honor the transformative power of intentional and nurturing practices. Through understanding the importance of self-care, designing personalized routines, and achieving a delicate balance with other commitments, individuals can foster a life of sustained well-being, resilience, and fulfillment.

CHAPTER 11

OVERCOMING COMMON HEALTH CHALLENGES

In the journey toward well-being, challenges are inevitable, yet surmountable. This chapter delves into strategies for overcoming common health challenges, addressing barriers to a healthy lifestyle, navigating setbacks, and building resilience for long-term well-being.

Addressing Barriers to a Healthy Lifestyle:

Barriers to a healthy lifestyle can emerge in various forms—time constraints, financial limitations, or even emotional hurdles. This section explores common barriers individuals face and provides practical insights into overcoming these challenges. From time management strategies to budget-friendly health practices, readers will discover actionable approaches that empower them to navigate and dismantle obstacles on their path to well-being.

The chapter emphasizes the importance of self-awareness in identifying and addressing personal barriers. By understanding individual challenges, individuals can adopt targeted strategies that make a positive impact on their health journey.

Strategies for Overcoming Setbacks:

Setbacks are not roadblocks but detours that offer opportunities for growth. This section guides readers in developing strategies for overcoming setbacks in their health journey. Whether facing a temporary lapse in healthy habits or encountering unexpected health issues, individuals will gain insights into resilience-building practices that help them bounce back stronger.

The chapter explores the role of self-compassion in navigating setbacks, emphasizing that acknowledging and learning from challenges contributes to long-term success. By reframing setbacks as learning experiences, individuals can build a resilient mindset that propels them forward on their health and well-being journey.

Building Resilience for Long-Term Well-being:

Resilience is the cornerstone of sustained well-being. This section delves into the art of building resilience—a skill that empowers individuals to navigate life's uncertainties and challenges with grace. From cultivating a positive mindset to fostering a support network, readers will discover strategies for enhancing their capacity to bounce back from adversity.

The chapter explores the connection between mindset and resilience, encouraging individuals to adopt a growth-oriented perspective. By viewing challenges as opportunities for personal development, individuals can build resilience that serves as a foundation for long-term well-being.

As we explore the strategies for overcoming common health challenges, let us embrace the notion that resilience is not the absence of challenges but the ability to navigate them with strength and adaptability. Through addressing barriers, navigating setbacks, and building resilience, individuals can cultivate a sustainable and resilient foundation for their health and well-being journey.

CHAPTER 12

HOLISTIC APPROACHES TO MENTAL HEALTH

Understanding mental health in a holistic context

In the tapestry of well-being, mental health is a vital thread intricately woven with the fabric of our overall health. This chapter explores holistic approaches to mental health, providing insights into understanding mental well-being in a broader context, introducing therapeutic practices, and promoting mental health awareness.

Understanding Mental Health in a Holistic Context:

Mental health extends beyond the absence of mental illness; it encompasses a state of balance, resilience, and emotional well-being. This section explores mental health in a holistic context, recognizing the interconnectedness of mind, body, and spirit. Readers will gain insights into the factors that influence mental well-being, from lifestyle choices and stress management to the quality of social connections.

The chapter emphasizes the importance of destigmatizing mental health and viewing it as an integral part of overall well-being. By understanding mental health holistically, individuals can adopt practices that promote emotional resilience, self-awareness, and a positive mindset.

Therapeutic Practices for Mental Well-being:

Holistic approaches to mental health incorporate a spectrum of therapeutic practices that extend beyond traditional interventions. This section introduces readers to therapeutic practices that nurture mental well-being, including mindfulness, meditation, expressive arts, and nature therapy. These practices offer individuals tools to manage stress, enhance self-reflection, and cultivate a deeper connection with themselves.

The chapter explores the role of nutrition, exercise, and sleep in supporting mental health, recognizing the profound impact of lifestyle choices on emotional well-being. By incorporating diverse therapeutic practices into daily life, individuals can foster a more resilient and balanced mental state.

Promoting Mental Health Awareness:

Promoting mental health awareness is a collective endeavor that contributes to breaking down barriers and fostering a supportive environment. This section explores strategies for promoting mental health awareness at individual and community levels. From open conversations and destigmatization efforts to educational initiatives, readers will discover practical approaches to raising awareness and creating a culture of understanding.

The chapter emphasizes the importance of empathy and active listening in promoting mental health awareness. By fostering a supportive and non-judgmental environment, individuals contribute to a culture that values mental well-being as an integral aspect of a flourishing life.

As we delve into holistic approaches to mental health, let us embrace the transformative potential of practices that nurture the mind, body, and spirit. Through understanding mental health in a holistic context, exploring therapeutic practices, and actively promoting mental health awareness, individuals contribute to a more compassionate and resilient society that values and prioritizes mental well-being.

CHAPTER 13

ENHANCING EMOTIONAL INTELLIGENCE

The role of emotional intelligence in health

Developing emotional awareness and regulation

Building healthier relationships through emotional intelligence

In the intricate landscape of well-being, emotional intelligence emerges as a guiding light—a skill that not only influences our mental and emotional health but also shapes the quality of our relationships. This chapter explores the pivotal role of emotional intelligence in health, guides readers in developing emotional awareness and regulation, and unravels the art of building healthier relationships through emotional intelligence.

The Role of Emotional Intelligence in Health:

Emotional intelligence is the keystone to navigating the complexities of human emotions and interactions. This section delves into the profound role of emotional intelligence in health, recognizing its impact on mental well-being, stress management, and overall life satisfaction. Readers will gain insights into how emotional intelligence serves as a compass for making informed decisions, building resilience, and fostering a positive mindset.

The chapter explores the interconnectedness of emotional intelligence with self-awareness, self-regulation, empathy, and interpersonal skills. By understanding the multifaceted nature of emotional intelligence, individuals can actively cultivate this skill to enhance their overall health and quality of life.

Developing Emotional Awareness and Regulation:

Emotional intelligence begins with self-awareness—a deep understanding of one's emotions and their impact. This section provides practical guidance on developing emotional awareness and regulation. From mindfulness practices that heighten present-moment awareness to techniques for identifying and managing emotions, readers will discover tools that empower them to navigate the intricate landscape of their own feelings.

The chapter emphasizes the importance of emotional regulation—a skill that enables individuals to respond to emotions in a constructive and balanced manner. By honing emotional awareness and regulation, individuals not only enhance their mental well-being but also lay the foundation for healthier relationships and effective communication.

Building Healthier Relationships Through Emotional Intelligence:

The fabric of our lives is woven with relationships, and emotional intelligence forms the thread that binds them. This section explores how emotional intelligence contributes to building healthier relationships. From empathetic communication to conflict resolution skills, readers will gain insights into the practices that foster understanding, trust, and connection.

The chapter acknowledges the role of emotional intelligence in cultivating a positive and supportive social environment. By applying emotional intelligence in interpersonal interactions, individuals contribute to the creation of relationships that promote mutual well-being and growth.

As we embark on the journey of enhancing emotional intelligence, let us recognize the transformative power of understanding and navigating our emotions. Through valuing the role of emotional intelligence in health, developing emotional awareness and regulation, and building healthier relationships, individuals can cultivate a more emotionally intelligent and fulfilling life.

CHAPTER 14

MINDFUL EATING FOR BETTER HEALTH

Exploring the concept of mindful eating

Benefits of mindful eating practices

Tips for incorporating mindfulness into mea

In the hustle of modern life, the simple act of eating can become a profound practice—a gateway to better health and well-being. This chapter explores the concept of mindful eating, delves into the benefits of mindful eating practices, and provides practical tips for incorporating mindfulness into meals.

Exploring the Concept of Mindful Eating:

Mindful eating is more than a dietary approach; it's a way of engaging with food and nourishing the body with intention. This section explores the concept of mindful eating, inviting readers to embrace a heightened awareness of the eating experience. From savoring flavors and textures to tuning into hunger and fullness cues, mindful eating is an invitation to be present in the moment and cultivate a deeper connection with food.

The chapter highlights the contrast between mindless eating, often driven by external cues and distractions, and the intentional and attuned approach of mindful eating. By understanding the principles of mindful eating, individuals can transform their relationship with food and pave the way for better health.

Benefits of Mindful Eating Practices:

The benefits of mindful eating extend beyond the nutritional value of food. This section explores the myriad advantages of incorporating mindful eating practices into daily life. From improved digestion and weight management to enhanced satisfaction and reduced stress, mindful eating contributes to a holistic sense of well-being.

The chapter also delves into the psychological benefits of mindful eating, such as a greater appreciation for food, increased self-awareness, and a reduction in emotional eating patterns. By savoring each bite and fostering a mindful approach to meals, individuals can derive both physical and mental nourishment.

Tips for Incorporating Mindfulness into Meals:

In the fast-paced rhythm of daily life, incorporating mindfulness into meals can be a transformative yet practical endeavor. This section provides readers with actionable tips for infusing mindfulness into their eating routines. From creating a serene eating environment to practicing gratitude for the food on the plate, readers will discover strategies for fostering a mindful approach to meals.

The chapter explores the role of mindful practices such as chewing slowly, paying attention to hunger and fullness cues, and avoiding distractions during meals. By embracing these tips, individuals can integrate mindfulness into their eating habits, promoting a more conscious and health-supportive relationship with food.

As we journey into the realm of mindful eating, let us recognize the transformative power of savoring each bite. Through exploring the concept of mindful eating, understanding its benefits, and incorporating mindfulness into meals, individuals can nourish not just their bodies but also their minds, fostering a more balanced and fulfilling relationship with food.

CHAPTER 15

EXPLORING HOLISTIC THERAPIES

Overview of complementary and alternative therapies

Integrating holistic therapies into your health routine

Consultation with healthcare professionals for holistic approaches

In the pursuit of comprehensive well-being, holistic therapies emerge as valuable tools, offering alternative approaches that consider the interconnectedness of mind, body, and spirit. This chapter provides an overview of complementary and alternative therapies, guides readers in integrating holistic therapies into their health routines, and underscores the importance of consulting with healthcare professionals for holistic approaches.

Overview of Complementary and Alternative Therapies:

Holistic therapies encompass a diverse range of practices that extend beyond conventional medicine. This section offers an overview of complementary and alternative therapies, exploring modalities such as acupuncture, herbal medicine, chiropractic care, massage therapy, and energy healing. Readers will gain insights into the principles, benefits, and potential applications of these approaches in promoting overall well-being.

The chapter emphasizes the holistic perspective that underlies these therapies, recognizing the importance of addressing not only symptoms but also the underlying imbalances that contribute to health issues. By understanding the principles of various holistic therapies, individuals can make informed decisions about integrating them into their health journey.

Integrating Holistic Therapies into Your Health Routine:

Holistic therapies can be seamlessly woven into a well-rounded health routine, complementing conventional approaches. This section provides practical guidance on integrating holistic therapies into daily life. From identifying specific health goals to researching and selecting appropriate therapies, readers will discover strategies for creating a personalized and effective holistic health plan.

The chapter explores the concept of synergy between conventional and holistic approaches, recognizing that an integrated approach can optimize health outcomes. By embracing a spectrum of therapeutic modalities, individuals can enhance their capacity to address health challenges and foster overall well-being.

Consultation with Healthcare Professionals for Holistic Approaches:

Collaboration with healthcare professionals is a cornerstone of responsible and effective holistic health practices. This section underscores the importance of consulting with healthcare professionals when incorporating holistic approaches into one's health routine. Whether seeking guidance on herbal supplements, exploring acupuncture for pain management, or considering energy healing for stress reduction, individuals can benefit from the expertise and insights of healthcare professionals.

As we delve into the exploration of holistic therapies, let us embrace the diversity of approaches that contribute to a holistic understanding of well-being. Through gaining an overview of complementary therapies, integrating them into a personalized health routine, and seeking professional guidance, individuals can embark on a journey that considers the richness of holistic health practices.

CHAPTE 17

SUSTAINABLE LIVING FOR HEALTH

In the quest for well-being, the connection between environmental consciousness and personal health is a powerful and symbiotic relationship. This chapter explores the intricate ties between environmental and personal health, provides insights into implementing eco-friendly practices for well-being, and guides readers in creating a sustainable and healthy lifestyle.

The Connection Between Environmental and Personal Health:

Our health is intimately woven into the health of the planet we inhabit. This section explores the profound connection between environmental and personal health, recognizing that the well-being of individuals is intricately linked to the health of the ecosystems around them. From air and water quality to the availability of nutritious food, the chapter delves into the environmental factors that directly impact personal health.

The chapter emphasizes the importance of understanding the broader ecological context in which individuals live. By recognizing the reciprocal relationship between personal and environmental health, readers can make informed choices that not only benefit their well-being but also contribute to the sustainability of the planet.

Implementing Eco-friendly Practices for Well-being:

Sustainable living involves mindful choices that prioritize both personal and environmental health. This section provides practical insights into implementing eco-friendly practices for well-being. From choosing sustainably sourced and organic foods to reducing waste and embracing energy-efficient habits, readers will discover actionable steps that contribute to a healthier lifestyle and a healthier planet.

The chapter explores the role of conscious consumerism, encouraging individuals to consider the environmental impact of their choices. By making eco-friendly decisions in areas such as transportation, clothing, and household products, individuals can align their lifestyle with principles of sustainability and well-being.

Creating a Sustainable and Healthy Lifestyle:

A sustainable and healthy lifestyle is a harmonious dance between personal wellness and environmental stewardship. This section guides readers in creating a lifestyle that embraces both these dimensions. From cultivating green spaces at home to engaging in outdoor activities that promote physical and mental health, readers will discover strategies for nurturing well-being while contributing to the sustainability of the environment.

The chapter also explores the concept of mindful consumption, inviting individuals to reflect on their habits and make intentional choices that align with their values. By adopting practices that promote sustainability and health, individuals can become catalysts for positive change, inspiring others to embrace a similar ethos.

As we explore the intersection of sustainable living and health, let us recognize the transformative potential of choices that honor both personal well-being and the health of the planet. Through understanding the connection between environmental and personal health, implementing eco-friendly practices, and creating a sustainable and healthy lifestyle, individuals can embark on a journey that not only enhances their well-being but also contributes to a thriving and resilient global ecosystem.

CHAPTER 18

CULTIVATING GRATITUDE FOR WELLNESS

Understanding the link between gratitude and health

Practices for cultivating a grateful mindset

Incorporating gratitude into daily life

In the intricate tapestry of well-being, gratitude emerges as a potent thread that weaves through the fabric of our mental, emotional, and physical health. This chapter explores the profound link between gratitude and health, provides practices for cultivating a grateful mindset, and guides readers in incorporating gratitude into their daily lives.

Gratitude is not merely a fleeting emotion; it is a transformative force with far-reaching implications for overall health. This section explores the scientific and psychological link between gratitude and well-being. From reducing stress and enhancing mental resilience to promoting positive emotions and improving sleep, the chapter delves into the multifaceted ways in which gratitude influences health.

Cultivating a grateful mindset is an art—a practice that transforms ordinary moments into sources of appreciation. This section provides practical insights into practices that nurture a grateful mindset. From keeping a gratitude journal to expressing appreciation to others, readers will discover a repertoire of techniques that foster a deep sense of gratitude.

The chapter explores the concept of mindful gratitude, encouraging individuals to savor the present moment and recognize the beauty in simple pleasures. By incorporating gratitude practices into daily routines, individuals can develop a habit of looking for and acknowledging the positive aspects of life.

Incorporating Gratitude into Daily Life:

Gratitude is not a fleeting emotion reserved for special occasions; it is a way of life. This section guides readers in incorporating gratitude into their daily lives, recognizing that small, consistent practices can yield profound results. From morning gratitude rituals to expressing thanks in challenging situations, readers will discover strategies for infusing daily life with the transformative power of gratitude.

As we explore the chapter on cultivating gratitude for wellness, let us recognize the profound impact of this simple yet transformative practice. Through understanding the link between gratitude and health, embracing practices that cultivate a grateful mindset, and incorporating gratitude into daily life, individuals can embark on a journey toward a more fulfilling, positive, and well-balanced existence.

CHAPTER 19

THE IMPACT OF TECHNOLOGY ON HEALTH

In the era of rapid technological advancement, the influence of technology on health is profound and multifaceted. This chapter explores the impact of technology on well-being, provides guidance on navigating the digital age for health, emphasizes the importance of balancing technology use, and addresses the management of screen time and its effects on mental health.

Navigating the Digital Age for Well-being:

Technology has become an integral part of modern life, offering unprecedented access to information, connectivity, and convenience. This section explores the challenges and opportunities presented by the digital age for well-being. From telemedicine and health-tracking apps to the potential impacts of social media on mental health, the chapter delves into the ways in which technology intersects with various aspects of our health.

The chapter emphasizes the importance of informed and intentional technology use, recognizing that harnessing the benefits of technology while mitigating its potential drawbacks requires mindfulness and a proactive approach.

Balancing Technology Use for Health Benefits:

Technology can be a powerful ally in the pursuit of health and well-being. This section provides insights into balancing technology use to maximize health benefits. From fitness apps that promote physical activity to mindfulness and meditation apps that support mental well-being, readers will discover ways to leverage technology for positive health outcomes.

The chapter explores the role of wearable devices, virtual health communities, and online resources that empower individuals to take an active role in managing their health. By adopting a strategic and balanced approach to technology use, individuals can integrate digital tools into their health routines for enhanced well-being.

Managing Screen Time and Its Effects on Mental Health:

While technology offers connectivity and information, excessive screen time can pose challenges to mental health. This section addresses the management of screen time and its effects on mental well-being. Readers will gain insights into the potential impacts of prolonged screen exposure, including digital eye strain, sleep disturbances, and the psychological effects of social media use.

The chapter provides practical strategies for managing screen time, establishing healthy digital habits, and creating boundaries for a more balanced relationship with technology. By fostering awareness of the potential drawbacks of excessive screen time, individuals can take proactive steps to prioritize their mental health in the digital age.

As we navigate the impact of technology on health, let us recognize its potential as a tool for empowerment. Through understanding the nuances of the digital age, balancing technology use for health benefits, and managing screen time with mindfulness, individuals can cultivate a harmonious relationship with technology that supports their overall well-being.

CHAPTER 20

EMBRACING A LIFELONG JOURNEY TO HEALTH

As we conclude this exploration of well-being, it's fitting to reflect on the seven proven ways to stay healthy and to underscore the significance of a continuous commitment to one's health. This final chapter serves as a recap of the key principles discussed throughout this book, emphasizing the importance of embracing a lifelong journey to health and offering encouragement for readers on their ongoing path to well-being.

Recap of the Seven Proven Ways to Stay Healthy:

Holistic Health: Recognizing the interconnectedness of mind, body, and spirit in fostering overall well-being.

Power of Nutrition: Understanding the impact of a balanced diet on health and tailoring nutritional choices to individual needs.

Exercise for a Healthy Body and Mind:
Incorporating a personalized fitness routine for physical
and mental well-being.

Role of Sleep in Well-being: Prioritizing quality
sleep and implementing practices for improved sleep
hygiene.

Stress Management Techniques: Recognizing the
effects of chronic stress and integrating mindfulness
and meditation practices into daily life.

Hydration for Vitality: Understanding the
significance of proper hydration and balancing beverage
choices for overall health.

Nurturing Social Connections: Valuing and
building meaningful relationships, combatting
loneliness through intentional connection.

Emphasizing the Importance of a Continuous
Commitment to Well-being:

Well-being is not a destination; it is a journey—one that
unfolds over a lifetime. This section emphasizes the

importance of maintaining a continuous commitment to one's health. Health is dynamic, and as circumstances change, so do the strategies needed to support well-being. It's an ongoing process of adaptation, learning, and refinement.

The chapter encourages readers to view setbacks not as failures but as opportunities for growth and learning. In a lifelong journey to health, every experience contributes to greater self-awareness and resilience. By embracing the ebb and flow of this journey, individuals can foster a mindset that promotes sustained well-being.

Encouragement for Readers to Embrace a Lifelong Journey to Health

In closing, this chapter serves as a source of encouragement for readers to wholeheartedly embrace their lifelong journey to health. It acknowledges the efforts made thus far and inspires a commitment to the ongoing process of self-discovery and well-being.

The journey to health is a personal and unique adventure. It requires resilience, patience, and a willingness to learn. This chapter encourages readers to celebrate their successes, no matter how small, and to

approach challenges with curiosity and an open heart.
It's a reminder that each day is an opportunity to make
choices that contribute to a healthier, more fulfilling life.

As we conclude this book, let us embark on the ongoing
journey to health with a sense of optimism,
determination, and a commitment to nurturing our
most precious asset—our well-being. May this journey
be a fulfilling and transformative exploration of the
boundless potential that lies within each of us.

CONCLUSION:

A HOLISTIC PATH TO LIFELONG WELL-BEING

In traversing the pages of "Seven Proven Ways to Stay Healthy: A Holistic Approach to Well-being," we've embarked on a journey through the intricate landscape of holistic health. We've explored the interconnected realms of mind, body, and spirit, uncovering seven proven ways to not only stay healthy but to thrive in the tapestry of our lives. As we conclude this exploration, let us reflect on the key insights that have woven the fabric of this holistic approach to well-being.

Holistic Health as the Foundation:

At the heart of our journey lies the recognition that health is a holistic endeavor, embracing every facet of our existence. We've delved into the profound interplay between mental and physical well-being, understanding that true health encompasses not just the absence of illness but a state of balance, resilience, and fulfillment.

The Seven Proven Ways:

Our exploration has unfolded through seven proven ways, each a pillar supporting the edifice of well-being:

Holistic Health: Recognizing the intricate dance of mind, body, and spirit in fostering overall well-being.

Power of Nutrition: Understanding the impact of a balanced diet on health and tailoring nutritional choices to individual needs.

Exercise for a Healthy Body and Mind: Incorporating a personalized fitness routine for physical and mental well-being.

Role of Sleep in Well-being: Prioritizing quality sleep and implementing practices for improved sleep hygiene.

Stress Management Techniques: Recognizing the effects of chronic stress and integrating mindfulness and meditation practices into daily life.

Hydration for Vitality: Understanding the significance of proper hydration and balancing beverage choices for overall health.

Nurturing Social Connections: Valuing and building meaningful relationships, combatting loneliness through intentional connection.

The Lifelong Journey:

Crucially, our exploration has not been a mere checklist but an invitation to a lifelong journey. Health is not a destination; it is a continuous commitment to self-discovery, growth, and well-being. Each principle, each practice, is a compass guiding us through the ebb and flow of life, helping us adapt, learn, and flourish.

Embracing Challenges and Celebrating Success:

As we conclude, let us remember that challenges are not roadblocks but stepping stones, and setbacks are opportunities for growth. Let us celebrate our successes, no matter how small, and approach each day with curiosity, optimism, and a commitment to making choices that nurture our health.

In the symphony of well-being, every aspect—nutrition, exercise, sleep, stress management, hydration, and social connections—plays a unique tune, harmonizing to create a melody of holistic health. May this book serve as a guide, a companion, and an inspiration on your lifelong journey to well-being—a journey where health is not just a destination but a way of life.

9 798874 006426